THE

LOW-FODMAP DIET

COOKBOOK

the low-fodmap diet cookbook for beginners: easy, healthy, quick recipes for your low-fodmap diet + days of helpful meal plans 2021

TABLE OF CONTENTS

BREAKFAST

Steamed Artichokes

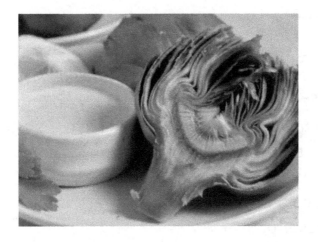

Preparation Time: 10 minutes

Cooking Time: 15 minutes

Servings: 4

Ingredients:

- 4 medium artichokes
- 1 lemon, halved
- 1 cup water

Directions:

1. To prepare the artichokes, use kitchen shears to trim the spiky tips off all the artichoke leaves. Pull off any tough leaves off the very bottom and use a paring knife to trim off the stem. Rub cut parts of the artichoke with the lemon to avoid discoloring.
2. Place a steamer insert or a rack in the pressure cooker pot.
3. Add the water to the pot. Arrange the artichokes in the pressure cooker, stacking them if necessary.
4. Lock lid and set the timer for 15 minutes at high pressure. When the timer is off, quick release the pressure, open the lid, and remove the artichokes with tongs. Serve hot or cool or use in another recipe.

Nutrition: Calories: 27 Carbs: 6g Fat: 0g Protein: 2g

Steamed Asparagus, Four Ways

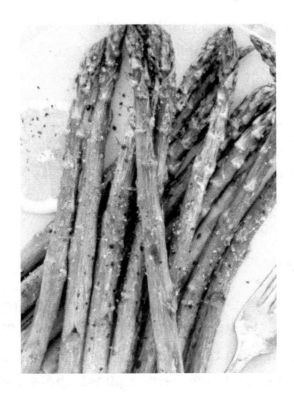

Preparation Time: 5 minutes

Cooking Time: 1 minute

Servings: 4

Ingredients:

- ½ cup water
- 1 pound asparagus, trimmed
- 2 tablespoons melted unsalted butter mixed
- ½ teaspoon freshly grated lemon zest
- 2 tablespoons champagne vinaigrette
- 1 tablespoon slivered almonds
- ¼ cup hollandaise sauce
- 1 tablespoon hazelnut oil
- 1 tablespoon chopped hazelnuts
- Salt and pepper

Directions:

1. Place a steamer insert in the pot of a pressure cooker. Add the water to the pot. Place the asparagus in the insert. If the stalks are too long, it's fine to lean them against the sides of the cooker.
2. Lock the lid then set the timer for 1 minute at high pressure. When the timer is off, quick release the pressure and open the lid. Transfer the asparagus to a plate.
3. Top or toss asparagus with one of the following:

4. 2 tablespoons melted unsalted butter mixed with ½ teaspoon freshly grated lemon zest
5. 2 tablespoons champagne vinaigrette and 1 tablespoon slivered almonds
6. ¼ cup hollandaise sauce
7. 1 tablespoon hazelnut oil and 1 tablespoon chopped hazelnuts. Season with salt and pepper.

Nutrition: Calories: 32 Carbs: 3g Fat: 1g Protein: 5g

Seasoned Bok Choy

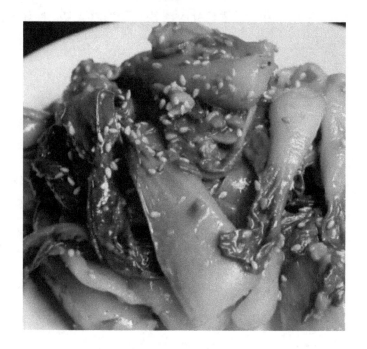

Preparation Time: 5 minutes

Cooking Time: 1 minute

Servings: 4

Ingredients:

- 1 cup water
- 4 baby bok choy heads, quartered lengthwise
- 1 tablespoon rice wine vinegar
- 1 teaspoon sesame oil
- 1 tablespoon toasted sesame seeds

Directions:

1. Place a steamer insert in the pot of a pressure cooker. Add the water to the cooker and mound the bok choy in the steamer.
2. Lock lid and set the timer for 1 minute at high pressure. When the timer is off, quick release the pressure and remove the cover, use transfer the bok choy to the platter or bowl.
3. In the bowl, whisk together the vinegar and sesame oil. Drizzle it over the bok choy. Sprinkle the sesame seeds over the bok choy and serve immediately.

Nutrition: Calories: 13 Carbs: 2g Fat: 0g Protein: 2g

Spicy Kale

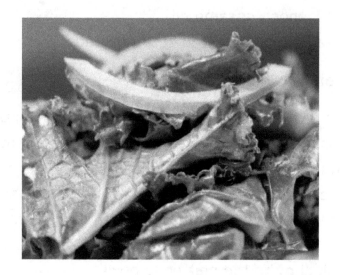

Preparation Time: 1 minute

Cooking Time: 5 minutes

Servings: 4

Ingredients:

- 1 tablespoon extra-virgin olive oil
- 2 garlic cloves, minced
- 1 kale bunch, stemmed and chopped or 1 (1-pound) bag chopped kale
- 1½ cups water
- 1 tablespoon red wine vinegar
- ½ teaspoon red pepper flakes
- ¼ teaspoon kosher salt

Directions:

1. With the pressure cooker on the sauté or brown setting, heat the olive oil. Add the garlic and sauté for 30 seconds, stirring constantly. Add the kale and water to the pressure cooker.
2. Then lock the lid and set the timer for 5 minutes at high pressure. When the timer is off, quick release the pressure, remove the lid, and toss the cooked greens with the vinegar, red pepper flakes, and salt. Serve hot.

Nutrition: Calories: 65 Carbs: 1g Fat: 1g Protein: 1g

Stewed Collard Greens

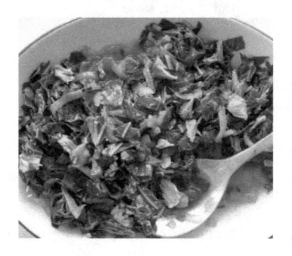

Preparation Time: 10 minutes

Cooking Time: 20 minutes

Servings: 4

Ingredients:

- 1 tablespoon vegetable oil
- 1 yellow onion, diced
- 1 collard greens bunch, roughly chopped
- 2 cups vegetable broth
- 1 teaspoon smoked paprika
- 1 tablespoon cider vinegar
- ½ teaspoon hot sauce
- ⅛ teaspoon kosher salt
- ⅛ teaspoon freshly ground black pepper

Directions:

1. With the pressure cooker on the sauté or brown setting, heat the vegetable oil until it shimmers. Sitr the onion and stir it frequently until it is softened and translucent, about 5 minutes. Add the collard greens, vegetable broth, and paprika.
2. Lock lid and set the timer for 20 minutes at high pressure. When the timer is off, naturally release it for 10 minutes. Then totally remove the lid after.
3. Stir in the vinegar, hot sauce, salt, and pepper. Serve hot.

4. To prepare the collard greens, rinse the leaves well by immersing them in a sink full of cool water. Fold leaves in half along the stem and use a chef's knife to cut away the toughest part of the stem. Then stack a few leaves at a time, roll them up into a cigar shape, and slice into wide ribbons. You can further chop the ribbons if desired.

Nutrition: Calories: 30 Carbs: 6g Fat: 0g Protein: 2g

Green Beans, Four Ways

Preparation Time: 10 minutes

Cooking Time: 2 minutes

Servings: 4

Ingredients:

- 1 cup water
- 4 pounds green beans, trimmed
- Salt and pepper
- 2 teaspoons extra-virgin olive oil
- 2 tablespoons finely grated parmesan cheese
- 1 cup mixed sliced mushrooms
- ¼ cup packaged fried onions
- ¼ cup toasted slivered almonds
- 2 teaspoons sesame oil over
- 1 tablespoon toasted sesame seeds

Directions:

1. Add the water to the pressure cooker pot. Place a steamer insert in the cooker. Place the beans in the steamer insert.
2. Lock lid and set the timer for 2 minutes at high pressure. When the timer is off, quick release the pressure and open the lid. Use tongs in trasferring the beans to a serving bowl.
3. Season the beans with one of the following:

4. Toss beans with salt, pepper, 2 teaspoons extra-virgin olive oil, and 2 tablespoons finely grated Parmesan cheese.
5. Place 1 tablespoon of unsalted butter on the hot beans and add salt and pepper. Toss with tongs to melt the butter and coat the beans. Sprinkle with ¼ cup toasted slivered almonds.
6. Drizzle 2 teaspoons sesame oil over the beans and add salt and pepper. Toss the beans with tongs to coat them with the oil. Sprinkle the toasted 1 tablespoon sesame seeds on the top of the beans.
7. Sauté 1 cup mixed sliced mushrooms in butter until softened, 6 to 7 minutes. Stir the mushrooms into the beans and add salt and pepper. Top with ¼ cup packaged fried onions.
8. To prepare green beans, break or trim the ends off each bean. You can do this by lining up a handful of beans on the cutting board and using a sharp knife to cut off all the ends at once.

Nutrition: Calories: 40 Carbs: 9g Fat: 0g Protein: 2g

Maple-Glazed Carrots

Preparation Time: 8 minutes

Cooking Time: 2 minutes

Servings: 4

Ingredients:

- 1 cup water
- 1 pound baby carrots
- 1½ tablespoons unsalted butter
- 1½ tablespoons pure maple syrup
- ¼ teaspoon kosher salt
- Pinch freshly ground black pepper
- 1 teaspoon fresh minced thyme

Directions:

1. Place the water and carrots in the pot of a pressure cooker.
2. Then lock the lid and set the timer for 2 minutes at high pressure. When timer is done, quick release the pressure, open the cooker, and switch to the brown setting.
3. Put the butter, maple syrup, salt, and pepper then sauté the carrots for 2 to 3 minutes or until the remaining liquid almost evaporates. Sprinkle with the fresh thyme. Serve hot or warm.

Nutrition: Calories: 110 Carbs: 0g Fat: 4g Protein: 1g

Beets, Two Ways

Preparation Time: 10 minutes

Cooking Time: 12 to 16 minutes

Servings: 4

Ingredients:

- 1 cup of water
- 1 pound medium-size beets, root, and stems trimmed
- For Version 1
- 2 tablespoons unsalted butter
- 2 tablespoons granulated sugar
- 2 tablespoons apple cider vinegar
- ⅛ teaspoon kosher salt
- Pinch freshly ground black pepper
- For Version 2
- 2 tablespoons unsalted butter
- ⅛ teaspoon kosher salt
- Pinch freshly ground black pepper
- ¼ cup finely grated Parmesan cheese
- 1 tablespoon minced fresh parsley

Directions:

1. Place a steamer insert or a rack in the pot of a pressure cooker. Add the water to the cooker. Place the beets on the steamer insert.

2. Lock on the lid then set the timer for 13 minutes at high pressure, less if the beets are very small. When timer is done, release the pressure and open the lid. Check the beets using fork; the fork should easily pierce the beets, which should still be firm but a bit of softness when squeezed. If they still seem very hard, like an uncooked potato, lock the lid back on and cook at high pressure for 3 more minutes.

3. When the beets are ready and cooked, remove from the cooker with tongs and let them rest until cool enough. Slip off the skins from the beets, they should come right off. Quarter the beets and slice into bite-size pieces.

4. To prepare version 1, remove the rack and pour the water out of the pressure cooker. With the setting on sauté or brown, melt the butter. Add the sugar and vinegar then stir until the sugar dissolves. Add the beets, and stir to coat them evenly with the vinegar mixture. Add the salt and pepper. Serve hot or warm. (Note: If you want to serve this recipe chilled, replace the butter with extra-virgin olive oil; otherwise, the butter will congeal.)

5. To prepare version 2, place the hot sliced beets into a bowl and toss with the butter, salt, and pepper. When the butter is already melted and it

coats the beets, add now the Parmesan and parsley and toss to distribute.

Nutrition: Calories: 154 Carbs: 20g Fat: 6g Protein: 5g

Crust less Spinach Quiche

Preparation Time: 10 minutes

Cooking Time: 5 hours

Servings: 6

Ingredients:

- Nonstick cooking spray
- 4 large eggs
- 1 cup half-and-half
- 1 cup shredded sharp Cheddar cheese
- 3 cups fresh baby spinach leaves
- 2 cups cubed ham
- ½ teaspoon salt
- ¼ teaspoon freshly ground black pepper

Directions:

1. Prepare a nonstick slow cooker and spray it with cooking spray.
2. In a large bowl, beat the eggs. Add the half-and-half, Cheddar cheese, spinach, ham, salt, and pepper and stir to combine. Pour the mixture into your slow cooker.
3. Cover your slow cooker. Cook for 5 hours on low or 3h hours on high.
4. Turn off the slow cooker and let it sit for 15 minutes before serving.

5. Empty a box of frozen spinach into a colander. Run warm water over the spinach until it's warm. Use a clean a paper towels or a towel to press down on the spinach and release as much water as possible.

Nutrition: Calories: 381 Total Fat: 27g Fat: 14g Cholesterol: 277mg Carbohydrates: 7g Fiber: 1g Protein: 27g

Blueberry-Coconut Quinoa

Preparation Time: 10 minutes

Cooking Time: 3 hours

Servings: 4

Ingredients:

- ¾ cup quinoa, rinsed and drained
- ¼ cup shredded unsweetened coconut
- 1 tablespoon honey
- 1 (13.5-ounce) can coconut milk
- 2 cups fresh blueberries

Directions:

1. Put the rinsed quinoa in the slow cooker. Sprinkle the coconut over the top and then drizzle with the honey.
2. Open the can of coconut milk. Stir until smooth and even in consistency. Pour over the quinoa.
3. Cover your slow cooker then cook for 3 hours on low.
4. Stir the quinoa, then scoop it into four serving bowls. Top each bowl with blueberries and serve.
5. If fresh blueberries are out of season or aren't available, you can easily substitute frozen blueberries, which are available year-round.

Nutrition: Calories: 468 Total Fat: 33g Carbohydrates: 43g Fiber: 7g Protein: 8g

Apple-Cinnamon Oatmeal

Preparation Time: 10 minutes

Cooking Time: 4 hours

Servings: 4

Ingredients:

- 1 cup steel-cut oats
- 1 tablespoon unsalted butter, melted
- 4 cups water
- ¼ cup brown sugar
- 1 teaspoon ground cinnamon
- ½ teaspoon salt
- 1 Granny Smith apple, peeled, cored, and chopped
- ½ cup milk

Directions:

1. Combine the steel-cut oats and butter in the slow cooker. Stir the oats until it is coated with the butter. Add the water, brown sugar, cinnamon, and salt.
2. Cover your slow cooker for it to cook for 4 hours in low.
3. Stir the chopped apple into the oatmeal. Scoop into four serving bowls and serve with a splash of milk.

Nutrition: Calories: 143 Total Fat: 4g Cholesterol: 10mg Sodium: 329mg Carbohydrates: 25g Fiber: 3g Protein: 3g

LUNCH

Roasted Maple Carrots

Preparation Time: 10 minutes

Cooking Time: 25 minutes

Servings: 3

Ingredients:

- 1 pound baby carrots
- 2 teaspoons fresh parsley, chopped
- 1 tablespoon Dijon mustard
- 2 tablespoons butter, melted
- 3 tablespoons maple syrup
- Pepper
- Salt

Directions:

1. Preheat the oven to 400 o F
2. In a large bowl, toss carrots with Dijon mustard, maple syrup, butter, pepper, and salt.
3. Transfer carrots to baking tray and spread evenly.
4. Roast carrots in preheated oven for 25-30 minutes. Serve and enjoy.

Nutrition: Calories: 177 Fat: 8.1g Protein: 1.3g Carbs: 26.2g

Sweet & Tangy Green Beans

Preparation Time: 10 minutes

Cooking Time: 15 minutes

Servings: 6

Ingredients:

- 1 ½ pounds green beans, trimmed
- 1 tablespoon maple syrup
- 2 tablespoons Dijon mustard
- 2 tablespoons rice wine vinegar
- ¼ cup olive oil
- ½ cup pecans, chopped
- Pepper
- Salt

Directions:

1. Preheat the oven to 400 o F
2. Place pecans on baking tray and toast in preheated oven for 5-8 minutes.
3. Remove from oven and let it cool.
4. Boil water in a large pot over high heat.
5. Add green beans in boiling water and cook for 4-5 minutes or until tender. Drain beans well and place in a large bowl.
6. Using a small bowl, whisk together oil, maple syrup, mustard, and vinegar.

7. Season beans with pepper and salt. Pour oil mixture over green beans.
8. Add pecans and toss well. Serve and enjoy.

Nutrition: Calories: 139 Fat: 10.4g Protein: 2.5g Carbs: 10.9g

Sautéed Carrots and Beans

Preparation Time: 10 minutes

Cooking Time: 10 minutes

Servings: 2

Ingredients:

- 2 cups green beans, trimmed
- 1 tablespoon fresh lemon juice
- 2 tablespoons butter
- 1 cup baby carrots, halved lengthwise
- 1 tablespoon olive oil
- Pepper
- Salt

Directions:

1. In a skillet over a medium-high heat, heat the olive oil.
2. Add carrots to the pan and cook for a minute.
3. Add green beans and cook until beans are just tender, season with pepper and salt.
4. Once vegetables are cooked then remove from pan and place on a plate.
5. Turn heat to medium-low and add butter in the same pan. Once butter is melted then add lemon juice and stir well.

6. Return vegetables to the pan and toss well to coat. Serve and enjoy.

Nutrition: Calories: 233 Fat: 18.7g Protein: 2.2g Carbs: 16g

Baked French toast

Preparation Time: 7 minutes

Cooking Time: 40 minutes

Servings: 6

Ingredients:

- 6 large eggs
- 2 cups lactose-free milk
- 2 tablespoons pure maple syrup
- 1 teaspoon pure vanilla extract
- 1/8 teaspoon sea salt
- 1 tablespoon ground cinnamon
- 6 slices gluten-free bread, lightly toasted

Directions:

1. Spray some coconut oil in your baking dish. In a medium bowl, whisk together eggs, milk, syrup, vanilla, salt, and cinnamon.
2. Arrange bread to fill the bottom of the baking dish—in 1 to 2 layers, trimming bread as necessary to fit. Pour liquid mixture evenly over the top. Cover and put overnight in the refrigerator.
3. On the next day, preheat oven to 375°F. Bake for 30 minutes or until egg mixture is completely set. Let stand 5 minutes before serving.

Nutrition: Calories: 230 Fat: 8g Protein: 12g Carbohydrates: 26g

Glazed Salmon

Preparation Time: 10 minutes

Cooking Time: 20 minutes

Servings: 4

Ingredients:

- ¼ cup gluten-free tamari
- 1 tablespoon almond butter
- 1 tablespoon pure maple syrup
- 2 teaspoons rice vinegar
- 2 teaspoons sesame oil
- 1 teaspoon blackstrap molasses
- 1/8 teaspoon ground ginger
- 12-ounce fillet of salmon

Directions:

1. Make the glaze: Mix all Ingredients except salmon in a small saucepan.
2. Transfer 2 tablespoons glaze to a small bowl.
3. Heat a charcoal grill, gas grill, or broiler to 350ºF. Grill or broil salmon, skin-side down, for 15 minutes, basting with the sauce in the small bowl.
4. While salmon is cooking, heat remaining glaze over medium-low heat for about 5 minutes to thicken.

5. When salmon is fully cooked, remove from heat, drizzle with heated glaze, and serve.

Nutrition: Calories: 190 Fat: 10g Protein: 19g Carbohydrates: 6g

DINNER

Eggplant Pasta

Preparation Time: 10 Minutes

Cooking Time: 25 Minutes

Servings: 4

Ingredients:

- 1 large eggplant, cut into cubes
- 2 cups tomato sauce
- 1 pound penne pasta, gluten-free
- 1/4 cup fresh parsley, chopped
- 1/4 cup fresh basil, chopped
- 1/2 teaspoon red chili flakes
- 2 tablespoons olive oil
- Kosher salt

Direction:

1. Ready to preheat your oven to 400 F/ 200 C.
2. Toss eggplant with 1 tablespoon oil and spread on a baking tray and roast for 25 minutes.
3. Cook pasta according to the packet instructions.
4. Heat remaining oil in a pan over medium heat.

5. Add tomato sauce, red pepper flakes, and eggplant and stir well.
6. Drain and wash well your pasta and add to the tomato mixture and stir well.
7. Garnish with parsley and basil. Serve and enjoy.

Nutrition: Calories: 457 Fat: 10.1g Protein: 16g Carbs: 78.2g

Ratatouille

Preparation Time: 10 Minutes

Cooking Time: 60 Minutes

Servings: 6

Ingredients:

- 1 large eggplant, steamed and sliced
- 4 medium zucchini, sliced
- 1 teaspoon dried basil
- 1/2 teaspoon dried oregano
- 1/4 teaspoon dried thyme
- 2 bell pepper, sliced
- 4 tomatoes, sliced
- 2 tablespoons olive oil

Directions:

1. Slice eggplant, zucchini, tomatoes, and bell pepper into 1/16-inch thick slices using a slicer.
2. Ready to preheat your oven to 400 F/ 200 C
3. Spray a baking dish with cooking spray and set aside.
4. Add all vegetable slices to a large bowl and season with salt and drizzle with oil.
5. Layer vegetable slices into the prepared dish and cover with foil.
6. Bake in preheated oven for 60 minutes.

7. Sprinkle with dried herbs. Serve and enjoy.

Nutrition: Calories: 123 Fat: 5.4g Protein: 3.9g Carbs: 18.6g

Sweet Potato Spinach Curry

Preparation Time: 10 Minutes

Cooking Time: 15 Minutes

Servings: 6

Ingredients:

- 3 ½ tablespoons olive oil
- ¼ teaspoon turmeric
- 1 teaspoon mustard seeds
- 1 tablespoon curry powder
- 1 tablespoon cumin seeds
- 1 pound spinach
- 1 large eggplant, peeled and cut into cube
- 1 large sweet potato, peeled and cut into cube
- 1 teaspoon salt

Directions:

1. Add water in a large pot and bring to boil.
2. Add spinach in boiling water and cook for 30 seconds. Drain well and chopped.
3. Heat oil in a pan over medium heat.
4. Add mustard seeds and sauté for 30 seconds.
5. Add cumin and cook for 1 minute.
6. Add sweet potatoes and cook for 5 minutes.

7. Add spinach, eggplant, curry powder, turmeric, and salt and cook for 7-8 minutes. Serve and enjoy.

Nutrition: Calories: 216 Fat: 13.8g Protein: 6g Carbs: 22.1g

Cabbage & Carrots

Preparation Time: 10 Minutes

Cooking Time: 10 Minutes

Servings: 2

Ingredients:

- 4 cups carrots, shredded
- 6 cups cabbage, shredded
- 1 teaspoon turmeric
- 1 tablespoon ginger, minced
- 1 tablespoon olive oil
- ¼ cup water
- ½ teaspoon sea salt

Directions:

1. In a pan heat your oil over medium-high heat.
2. Add cabbage and cook for 8 minutes.
3. Add carrots and cook for 2-3 minutes.
4. Add turmeric, ginger, water, and salt and stir well.
5. Turn heat to low and cook until carrots are softened. Serve and enjoy.

Nutrition: Calories: 119 Fat: 3.8g Protein: 2.7g Carbs: 20.8g

Quinoa Vegetable Salad

Preparation Time: 10 Minutes

Cooking Time: 20 Minutes

Servings: 8

Ingredients:

- 1 cup quinoa, uncooked
- 1 tablespoon vinegar
- 2 teaspoons sesame oil
- ¼ cup soy sauce, low sodium
- 2 green onions, green part only chopped
- ½ cup bell pepper, chopped
- 1 cup zucchini, chopped
- 1 cup red cabbage, shredded
- ½ teaspoon ground ginger
- 2 cups water
- Salt

Directions:

1. Adding your quinoa and water in a saucepan and bring to boil over medium-high heat.
2. Turn heat to low and simmer for 15 minutes.
3. Transfer quinoa in a mixing bowl.
4. Add cabbage, green onion, bell pepper, zucchini, and salt in quinoa and mix well.

5. In a small bowl, whisk together ginger, vinegar, sesame oil, and soy sauce and pour over quinoa mixture. Serve and enjoy.

Nutrition: Calories: 101 Fat: 2.5g Protein: 3.9g Carbs: 16.1g

Herb Quinoa

Preparation Time: 10 Minutes

Cooking Time: 15 Minutes

Servings: 2

Ingredients:

- 1 cup quinoa, rinsed
- 2 cups water
- 1 teaspoon lemon zest, grated
- 1 ½ teaspoon fresh mint, chopped
- 1 tablespoon fresh cilantro, chopped
- 1 tablespoon fresh basil, chopped
- ½ teaspoon salt

Directions:

1. In your pan put some water and bring to boil.
2. Adding your quinoa and salt to the boiling water. Cover and simmer over low heat for 12-15 minutes.
3. Remove saucepan from heat.
4. Fluff quinoa with a fork and add in a large bowl.
5. Add remaining ingredients into the quinoa and stir well. Serve and enjoy.

Nutrition: Calories: 315 Fat: 5.2g Protein: 12.1g Carbs: 54.9g

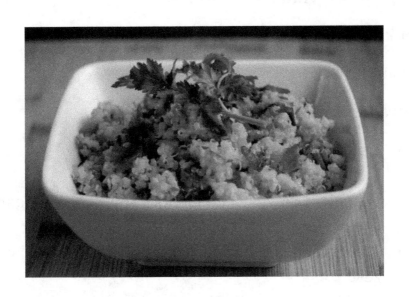

VEGETABLES, AND SALADS RECIPES

Cheesy Broccoli & Zucchini Fritters

Preparation Time: 10 Minutes

Cooking Time: 15 Minutes

Servings: 3

Ingredients:

- 2 cup broccoli florets, steamed
- 1 cup zucchini, grated
- ½ cup Colby, Cheddar or soy-based vegan cheese, grated
- 2 teaspoon fresh lime juice & ½ teaspoon lime zest
- 3 tablespoons low FODMAP milk
- ½ cup gluten-free all-purpose flour
- ¼ teaspoon salt
- ¼ teaspoon black pepper
- 1 egg, beaten
- 2 tablespoons garlic-infused oil
- ¼ cup mayonnaise

Directions:

1. Mash the steamed broccoli. Set aside.
2. Whisk together the egg, milk, and 1 tablespoon of garlic-infused oil in a small bowl.
3. Mix in the flour, salt, and black pepper until thick and smooth.
4. Now add the steamed broccoli, zucchini, and cheese.
5. Heat remaining oil in a large skillet. Add quarter cup measures of the fritters and flatten own with a spatula.
6. Cook the fritters for 3-4 minutes each side.
7. Mix the lime juice and zest with the mayonnaise. Serve alongside the fritters.

Nutrition: Calories 310 Fat 17g Carbs 28g Protein 11g

Bacon, Sweet Potato & Kale Hash

Preparation Time: 10 Minutes

Cooking Time: 15 Minutes

Servings: 3

Ingredients:

- 1 sweet potato, peeled and diced into ¼ -inch cubes
- 3 rashers bacon,
- 1 cup kale, chopped with stalks removed
- 1 bell pepper, diced
- 3 eggs
- 1 tablespoon vegetable oil
- Salt and freshly ground pepper to taste

Directions:

1. Preheat your oven to 400°F.
2. Fry the bacon until crisp in a large ovenproof skillet. Remove from the pan and set aside.
3. Arrange the sweet potato in the skillet and cook undisturbed until brown on one side.
4. Flip the sweet potato cubes over and brown on the other side.
5. Add the kale and bell peppers and stir to soften the vegetables. Season with salt and pepper.
6. Make wells in the mixture and crack in the eggs.

7. Transfer the skillet to the oven and cook for approximately 10 minutes depending on how you like your eggs.
8. Serve with bacon crumbled over the top.

Nutrition: Calories 161 Fat 9g Carbs 14g Protein 9g

Maple, Orange & Thyme Glazed Baby Carrots

Preparation Time: 20 minutes

Cooking Time: 20 minutes

Servings: 4

Ingredients:

- 2 cup baby carrots, trimmed and scrubbed
- 2½ tablespoons butter, salted
- ½ cup freshly squeezed orange juice
- 1 teaspoon orange zest
- 1 tablespoon thyme, chopped
- ⅓ Cup maple syrup
- ½ teaspoon salt
- ½ teaspoon black pepper
- 1 tablespoon mustard

Directions:

1. Melt the butter in a large non-stick skillet pan with a close-fitting lid.
2. Add carrots, maple syrup, orange juice, zest, and the salt and pepper.
3. Bring to the boil and cover with the lid. Reduce the heat and cook for about 4 minutes.
4. Uncover and cook for a further 15 minutes.
5. Serve garnished with fresh thyme.

Nutrition: Calories 185 Fat 10g Carbs 22g Protein 1g

Glazed Ham

Preparation Time: 30 minutes

Cooking Time: 4 hours

Servings: 25

Ingredients

- 1 16 pound ham on the bone
- ⅓ Cup freshly squeezed orange juice
- ⅓ Cup brown sugar
- ⅓ Cup maple syrup
- 1 tablespoon Dijon mustard
- 30 whole cloves

Directions:

1. Preheat the oven to 300ºF.
2. Line a large baking tray with two layers of baking paper.
3. Place the ham in the baking tray and place in the oven for 10 minutes to warm the skin.
4. Whisk together the maple syrup, brown sugar, orange juice, and dijon mustard in a small bowl.
5. Remove the ham from the oven and increase the oven temperature to 340ºF.

6. Make a cut around the ham using a sharp knife then use your fingers to peel away the rind and fat.
7. Score the ham in a diamond pattern, and stud the centers of the diamonds with cloves. Baste with glaze and place into the oven.
8. Bake for approximately 4 hours basting every half hour.

Nutrition: Calories 495 Fat 18g Carbs 6g Protein 72g

Beef Burgers with BBQ Sauce

Preparation Time: 15 minutes

Cooking Time: 30 minutes

Servings 4

Ingredients

- 1lb lean ground beef
- ¼ cup green scallions, green tips only, finely chopped
- ¼ cup gluten-free breadcrumbs
- 3 medium carrots, peeled & cut into chunks
- ½ teaspoon dried thyme
- 1 teaspoon dried oregano
- 1 teaspoon dried basil
- 1 tablespoon Worcestershire sauce
- Salt & pepper
- 1½ teaspoon vegetable oil
- Salt & freshly ground black pepper
- 1 large egg, lightly beaten

Directions:

1. Preheat the oven to 410ºF.
2. Place the carrots into a roasting tray and toss with oil. Bake for approximately 30 minutes.
3. In a large bowl, mix the lean ground beef, scallion's tips, breadcrumbs, dried herbs,

Worcestershire sauce, beaten egg, and salt and pepper.

4. Divide the mixture evenly into 8 patties.
5. Fry the patties for 7 minutes each side.
6. Serve the burgers on toasted the gluten-free buns if desired with shredded lettuce, tomatoes, and cucumber.

Nutrition: Calories 613 Fat 23g Carbs 62g Protein 40g

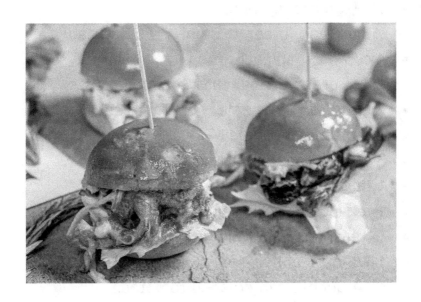

Spaghetti Bolognese

Preparation Time: 40 minutes

Cooking Time: 40 minutes

Servings: 4

Ingredients

- 1lb lean ground beef
- ½ cup leek, green tips only, thinly sliced
- 4 cup baby spinach, roughly chopped
- 1 cup green beans, cut into small pieces
- 2 large carrots, peeled & cut into sticks
- 1 tablespoon olive oil
- 3 tablespoons tomato paste
- 1 teaspoon dried oregano
- 1 teaspoon dried basil
- ½ teaspoon dried thyme
- 12 ounces gluten-free spaghetti
- 1 14 ounces can crushed tomatoes
- Salt & freshly ground pepper

Directions:

1. Cook the beef until browned in a large skillet.
2. Add canned tomatoes, tomato paste, leek tips, baby spinach, and herbs and allow to simmer for 20 minutes. Add salt and pepper to taste.

3. Cook the pasta according to the instructions on the packet.
4. Cook green beans and carrots in boiling water until tender.
5. Serve the Bolognese on a bed of spaghetti with the cheese on top and a side of vegetables.

Nutrition: Calories 642 Fat 19g Carbs 82g Protein 40g

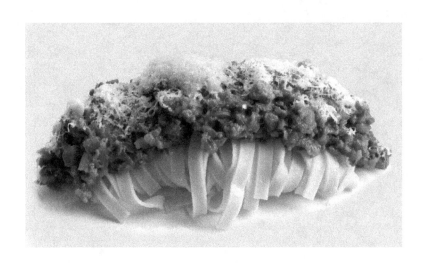

Espresso Rib eye

Preparation time: 15 minutes

Cooking time: 10 minutes

Servings: 4

Ingredients:

- 1 2 pounds bone-in rib-eye steak, about 1½ inches thick
- 1 tablespoon salted butter
- 1½ tablespoon vegetable oil
- 1½ teaspoons flaky sea salt
- 1 teaspoons black pepper
- ⅓ Cup instant espresso granules
- 2 teaspoons ancho chili powder

Directions:

1. Preheat the oven to 450°F.
2. Rub both sides of the steak with ½ tablespoon of the oil, and season with salt and pepper.
3. Rub both sides of the steak with the espresso granules and chili powder. Set aside for 30 minutes.
4. Place an ovenproof skillet in the oven until hot for 10 minutes.
5. Remove the hot skillet from the oven and add the remaining oil to the pan.

6. Place the steak in the skillet and leave to cook for 3 minutes.
7. Flip the steak and cook, undisturbed, again for a further 3 minutes.
8. Use tongs to hold the edges of the steak to the pan. Cook for an additional 6 minutes this way.
9. Place the steak in the skillet in the oven for 6 to 8 minutes for medium-rare.
10.　　Remove the steak from the skillet; top with the butter, and let rest for 10 minutes before serving.

Nutrition: Calories 552 Fat 46g Carbs 3g Protein 8g

Sweet Potato & Lamb Fritters with Salad

Preparation Time: 20 Minutes

Cooking Time: 20 Minutes

Servings: 4

Ingredients:

- 10 ounces sweet potato, peeled & diced
- 10 ounces potato, peeled & diced
- 1 pound lean ground lamb
- 1 cup green scallions, green tips only, finely chopped
- 1 cup fresh cilantro, chopped
- 1 tablespoon garlic-infused oil
- 1 tablespoon crushed ginger
- 2 teaspoons soy sauce
- 1 tablespoon oyster sauce

Directions:

1. Preheat the oven to 350ºF.
2. Boil the sweet potatoes and potatoes until tender. Then roughly mash with a fork. Set aside.
3. Heat the oil in a large skillet and fry the lamb.
4. Add ginger, spring onion tips, soy sauce, oyster sauce, and fresh cilantro.

5. Mix the lamb with the potato mixture in a large bowl.
6. Scoop out quarter cup measures of mixture and shape into fritters. Place the fritters on a baking pan lined with parchment paper.
7. Place in the oven and bake for 10 minutes each side, until golden brown.
8. Serve with a salad made of lettuce, grated carrot, tomatoes, and cucumbers.

Nutrition: Calories 465 Fat 27g Carbs 33g Protein 24g

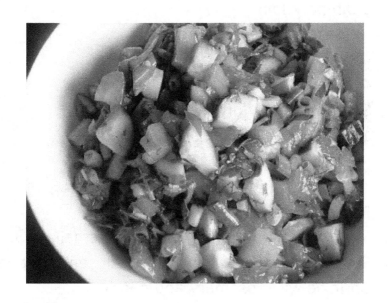

Pork Loin with Maple Mustard Sauce

Preparation Time: 10 Minutes

Cooking Time: 60 Minutes

Servings: 12

Ingredients:

- 1 3lb pork loin
- ½ teaspoon smoked paprika
- 4 tablespoons maple syrup
- 4 tablespoons wholegrain mustard
- Salt and freshly ground black pepper
- 1 teaspoon dry rosemary, crushed

Directions:

1. Preheat oven to 350°F.
2. Mix maple syrup and mustard in a small bowl.
3. Season the pork loin with salt and pepper. Sprinkle with rosemary and paprika.
4. Place pork loin in roasting pan and brush with maple mustard sauce.
5. Roast for about 1 hour, basting with extra sauce halfway through cooking.

Nutrition: Calories 271 Fat 17g Carbs 7g Protein 22g

POULTRY RECIPES

Moroccan Chicken

Preparation Time: 8 hours

Cooking Time: 16 minutes

Servings: 4

Ingredients:

- 2 tablespoons olive oil
- 2 teaspoons ground paprika
- 1 teaspoon ground cumin
- ½ teaspoon ground coriander
- ½ teaspoon ground turmeric
- ¼ teaspoon ground ginger
- 1/8 teaspoon cayenne pepper
- 1 package 20-oz boneless and skinless chicken breasts
- Salt and pepper to taste

Directions:

1. In a bowl, combine all ingredients except for the chicken.

---

2. Transfer your chicken breasts in a Ziploc bag and pour in the sauce. Allow to marinate in the fridge for at least 8 hours.
3. Heat the grill to medium and remove the chicken from the marinade.
4. Grill the chicken for 8 minutes on each side until fully cooked.

Nutrition: Calories 237 Fat 10.2g Carbs 1.2g Protein 32.2g

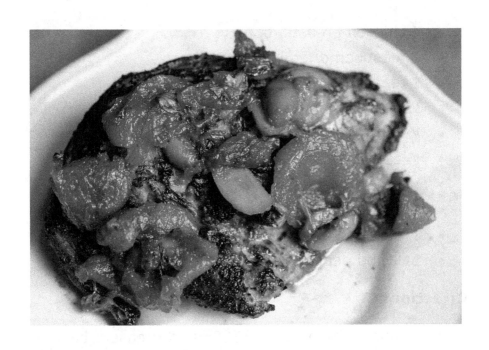

Chicken Pub Rub

Preparation Time: 10 minutes

Cooking Time: 30 minutes

Servings: 4

Ingredients:

- 4 chicken breasts, bone in
- 1 teaspoon dried basil
- 1 teaspoon dried rosemary
- ½ teaspoon mustard powder
- ½ teaspoon paprika
- ½ teaspoon dried thyme
- ¼ teaspoon celery seed
- 1/8 teaspoon ground cumin
- 1/8 teaspoon cayenne pepper
- Salt and pepper to taste

Directions:

1. Preheat the oven to 3500F and grease a baking dish.
2. Mixed all the ingredients in a bowl and mix until the chicken is coated with the condiments.
3. Place the chicken in the baking dish. Get a foil and cover to prevent the chicken from drying out.

4. Cook for 30 minutes until the internal temperature of the chicken reaches 2050F.

Nutrition: Calories 502 Fat 26.9g Carbs 0.5g Protein 60.6g

Thai Green Curried Chicken

Preparation Time: 10 minutes

Cooking Time: 15 minutes

Servings: 6

Ingredients:

- 2 stalks lemon grass
- 4 green chilies
- 6 spring onions, green part only
- 1 tablespoon grated ginger
- ½ cup fresh coriander
- ½ cup fresh basil
- 1 teaspoon ground cumin
- 1 teaspoon fish sauce
- Zest from one lemon
- 2 tablespoons coconut oil
- 1 ½ chicken breasts, cut into bite-sized pieces
- 1 can coconut milk
- 2 sweet peppers, cut into strips
- ¾ cup baby corn, sliced

- Salt and pepper
- ½ cup water

Directions:

1. In a food processor, place the lemon grass, green chilies, onions, ginger, coriander, basil, ground cumin, fish sauce, and lemon zest. Pulse until a smooth paste is formed. Set aside.
2. Using a deep pan heat your oil over medium flame and sauté the green paste made earlier. Stir for 30 seconds to a minute.
3. Stir in the chicken breasts and season with salt and pepper to taste. Cook for 5 minutes.
4. Bring to boil your poured coconut milk and water. Once boiled, stir in the sweet peppers and baby corn. Continue cooking for another 5 minutes.

Nutrition: Calories 195 Fat 9.4g Carbs 15.1g Protein 9.4g

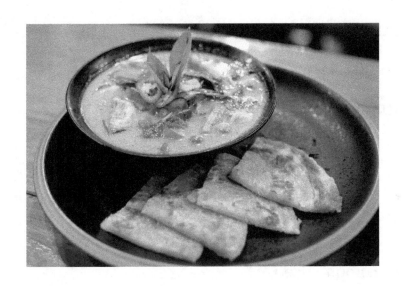

SIDE DISHES, SAUCES AND DIPS RECIPES

Chive and Onion-Infused Dip

Preparation Time: 10 minutes

Cooking Time: 5 minutes

Servings: 10

Ingredients:

- Onion chunks
- 3 tablespoons olive oil
- Mayonnaise
- Parsley, chopped
- Chives, dried
- Lemon juice

Directions:

1. Fry the onion in olive oil for about 4 minutes.
2. Once fragrant, remove all of the onion chunks from the oil. Set aside to cool.
3. Place all of the ingredients in a bowl and mix well. Add more lemon juice, parsley and/or chives if desired.

4. Refrigerate for 30 minutes.

Nutrition: Calories 82 Fat 7.8g Protein 0.4g
Carbohydrates 2.9g

Traditional Hummus

Preparation Time: 15 minutes

Cooking Time: 12 minutes

Servings: 8

Ingredients:

- 400 grams canned chickpeas, rinsed, drained and skinned
- 3 tablespoons water
- 2 tablespoons tahini
- ½ teaspoon salt
- 1 tablespoon olive oil
- 2 tablespoons lemon juice
- ½ teaspoon cumin, ground
- 2 teaspoons garlic-infused oil

Directions:

1. Put tahini and lemon juice in a food processor. Blend until smooth.
2. Add remaining ingredients into the tahini mixture. Blend until desired consistency is obtained.
3. Refrigerate for 30 minutes.

Nutrition: Calories: 83 Fat: 7.9g Carbs: 1.9g Protein: 2.3g

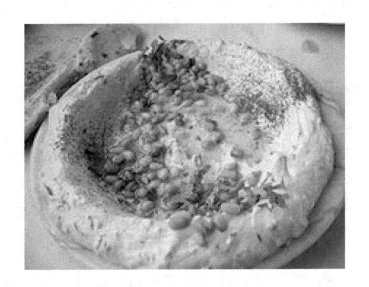

Sunflower Seed Butter

Preparation Time: 15 minutes

Cooking Time: 40 minutes

Servings: 26

Ingredients:

- 40 grams raw sunflower seeds, hulled
- 1 tablespoon pure maple syrup
- 1 tablespoon coconut oil ¼ teaspoon salt

Directions:

1. Set the oven to 190 degrees Celsius.
2. Distribute the sunflower seeds evenly on a roasting tray lined with baking paper.
3. Bake for 20 minutes. Stir the seeds every 5 minutes throughout the cook. Set aside to cool.
4. Transfer the seeds to a food processor. Blitz the seeds for 20 minutes. Remember to stop every now and then to scrape the sides of the food processor and break down the lumps in the mixture.
5. Add the remaining ingredients once butter is creamy and smooth. Blitz for another minute.

Nutrition: Calories: 101 Fat: 8.9g Carbs: 3.8g Protein: 3.4g

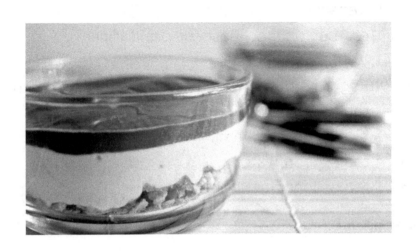

Pumpkin and Roast Pepper Hummus

Preparation Time: 15 minutes

Cook Time: 15 minutes

Servings: 15

Ingredients:

- 200 grams chickpeas, rinsed and drained
- ½ teaspoon cumin, ground
- 1 red bell pepper, deseeded and sliced
- 1 ½ teaspoon paprika
- 400 grams buttercup squash, peeled and sliced
- 3 tablespoons lemon juice
- 2 tablespoons olive oil
- 4 tablespoon water
- 1 tablespoons garlic-infused oil

Directions:

1. Set the oven to 190 degrees Celsius.
2. Put bell pepper strips in a tray and sprinkle olive oil on top. Roast for 10 minutes.
3. Place squash and water in a bowl. Set microwave on high and heat it while covered for 9 minutes.
4. Put the remaining ingredients in a food processor. Add squash and bell pepper. Season to taste.
5. Blend until smooth.

Nutrition: Calories: 59 Fat: 3.4g Carbs: 6.3g Protein: 1.6g

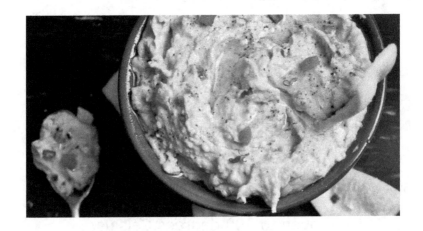

Pumpkin Dip

Preparation Time: 10 minutes

Cook Time: 40 minutes

Servings: 8

Ingredients:

- 500 grams buttercup squash, peeled and sliced
- ½ tablespoon garlic-infused oil
- 1 tablespoon canola oil
- 2 tablespoons lemon juice
- 2 tablespoons mayonnaise
- ½ teaspoon paprika
- 1 tablespoon fresh rosemary, chopped
- Salt and pepper

Directions:

1. Set the oven to 200 degrees Celsius.
2. Put pumpkin pieces in a tray and drizzle with oil. Season to taste.
3. Roast for 30 minutes then set aside for 10 minutes to cool.
4. Transfer the roast pumpkin to a food processor. Add remaining ingredients and blend until smooth.

Nutrition: Calories: 58 Fat: 3.8g Carbs: 6.2g Protein: 1.3g

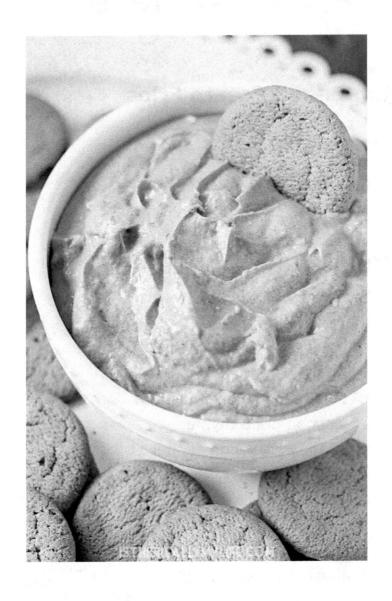

SNACKS, DESSERT AND APPETIZER RECIPES

Cajun Baked Potato Fries

Preparation Time:

Cooking Time: 35 minutes

Servings: 2

Ingredients:

- 2 tablespoons olive oil
- 2 large sweet potatoes
- 1 ½ teaspoon garlic powder
- 1 ½ teaspoon dried oregano
- 1 ½ teaspoon smoked paprika
- 1 teaspoon dried thyme
- ¼ teaspoon cayenne pepper
- ½ teaspoon salt
- ¼ teaspoon black pepper

Directions:

1. Preheat the oven to 425F.

2. Cut sweet potatoes into match sticks. Transfer to two baking sheets and add olive oil. Mix with seasonings, sugar and toss well.
3. Arrange fries in a single layer and bake for 15 minutes. Flip and bake for 15 more minutes.
4. Remove and serve.

Nutrition: Calories: 197 Fat: 13.7g Carbs: 18.2g Protein: 1.8g

Spicy Smoky Kale Chips

Preparation Time: 15 minutes

Cooking Time: 14 minutes

Servings: 4

Ingredients:

- 1 bunch kale, rinsed and dried
- 1 tablespoon chili flakes
- Olive oil
- Salt, to taste

Directions:

1. Preheat the oven to 350F.
2. Trim kale leaves. Cut in half. Add to a bowl.
3. Add 1 tablespoon olive oil and toss. Add chili flakes and salt. Transfer to a baking sheet lined tray and place in a single layer. Bake for 14 minutes. Serve.

Nutrition: Calories: 115 Fat: 5g Carbs: 3g Protein: 6g

Salmon Mini Cakes

Preparation Time: 15 minutes

Cook Time: 40 minutes

Servings: 6-8

Ingredients:

- 2 tablespoons olive oil
- 2 large baking potatoes
- 1 egg yolk
- 1/2 lemon juice and zest
- 1 tablespoon parsley, chopped
- 2 tablespoon gluten free flour
- 1 teaspoon black pepper
- 5 ounces smoked salmon trimmings

Directions:

1. Microwave potatoes for 10 minutes on high. Let rest for 5 minutes.
2. Crashed the potato flesh in a bowl and let cool. Add lemon juice, olive oil and lemon zest. Add egg and parsley, stir well to combine.
3. Shape mini cakes. Refrigerate for 10 minutes.
4. Dip each cake into flour and fry over low heat for 3 minutes per side in little oil. Drain and serve with salmon and parsley.

Nutrition: Calories: 321 Fat: 15g Carbs: 5g Protein: 3g

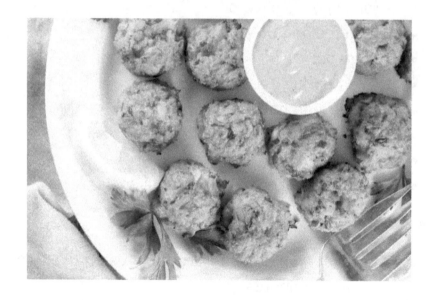

Spiced Quinoa with Almonds and Feta

Preparation Time: 15 minutes

Cooking Time: 20 minutes

Servings: 4

Ingredients:

- 1 ½ cups quinoa, rinsed
- 1/2 teaspoon turmeric
- 1 tablespoon olive oil
- 1 teaspoon ground coriander
- 1/2 cup almonds, toasted and flaked
- 1 cup feta cheese, crumbled
- 1/2 lemon juice
- A handful parsley, chopped

Directions:

1. Heat oil in a pan. Add spices and fry for 1 minute.
2. Add quinoa and fry for 1 more minute. Add 2 1/2 cup boiling water and cook for 15 minutes.
3. Let cool and add remaining ingredients. Stir well and serve.

Nutrition: Calories: 321 Fat: 15g Carbs: 5g Protein: 3g

Salmon and Spinach with Tartar Cream

Preparation Time:

Cooking Time: 15 minutes

Servings: 2

Ingredients:

- 2 salmon fillets, skinless
- 1 teaspoon vegetable oil
- 1 1/8 cup spinach
- 2 tablespoon crème fraiche
- 1 teaspoon caper, drained
- 1/2 lemon juice
- 2 tablespoon flat-leaf parsley, chopped
- Lemon wedges

Directions:

1. Heat oil in a pan. Season salmon well. Fry salmon for 4 minutes per side. Transfer to a plate and let rest.
2. Add parsley leaves into the pan, season and cover and wilt for 1 minute. Add spinach onto plates and top with salmon.
3. Heat crème fraiche in the pan with lemon juice, capers and parsley. Season well to taste.

4. Add the sauce over the fish and serve with lemon wedges.

Nutrition: Calories: 321 Fat: 15g Carbs: 5g Protein: 3g

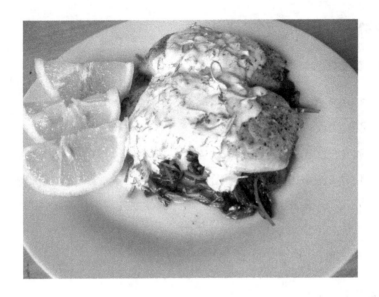

DRINKS

Oatmeal Cookie Breakfast Smoothie

Preparation Time: 2 Minutes

Cooking Time: 0 Minutes

Servings: 1

Ingredients:

- 1 yellow banana, peeled and sliced
- ¾ cup almond milk
- ¼ cup ice
- 1/8 tablespoon vanilla
- ½ teaspoon cinnamon powder
- 2 tablespoons rolled oats
- A dash of ground nutmeg

Directions:

1. Place all ingredients in a blender. Pulse until smooth. Serve immediately.

Nutrition: Calories: 303 kcal Fat: 7.8 g Carbs: 60 g Protein: 5.5 g

Green Kiwi Smoothie

Preparation Time: 3 Minutes

Cooking Time: 0 Minutes

Servings: 2

Ingredients:

- 1 cup seedless green grapes
- 1 kiwi, peeled and chopped
- 2 tablespoons water
- 8 inches cucumber, cut into chunks
- 2 cups baby spinach
- 1 ½ cups ice cubes
- 1 green apple, peeled and cored

Directions:

1. Place all ingredients in a blender. Pulse until the mixture becomes smooth. Serve immediately.

Nutrition: Calories: 132 kcal Fat: 1 g Carbs: 33 g Protein: 3 g

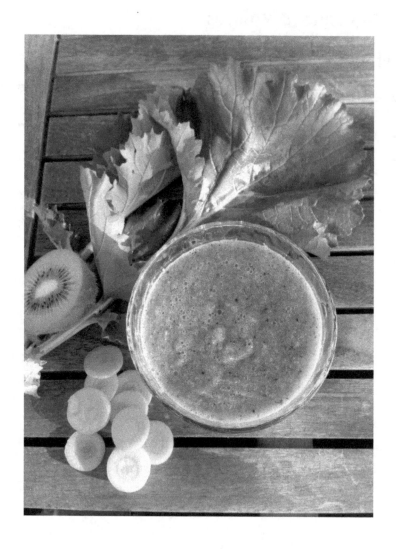

Pumpkin Smoothie

Preparation Time: 2 Minutes

Cooking Time: 0 Minutes

Servings: 1

Ingredients:

- ¼ cup pumpkin puree
- ½ cup coconut milk
- ¼ teaspoon pumpkin pie spice
- 1 tablespoon maple syrup
- ½ cup crushed ice
- A pinch of cinnamon
- ½ frozen medium ripe bananas, peeled and sliced

Directions:

1. Place all ingredients in a blender except for the cinnamon. Blend until smooth. Put into glasses and sprinkle with cinnamon before serving.

Nutrition: Calories: 695 Fat: 37.7 g Carbs: 52.3 g Protein: 14.3 g

Chocolate Sesame Smoothie

Preparation Time: 2 Minutes

Cooking Time: 0 Minutes

Servings: 1

Ingredients:

- 1 tablespoon sesame seeds
- 2 teaspoons unsweetened raw cocoa powder
- Flesh from 1/8 slice of avocado
- 1 tablespoon maple syrup
- 1 cup coconut milk
- ½ cup ice
- Half of a medium banana, peeled and sliced

Directions:

1. Place all ingredients in a blender. Pulse until smooth. Pour in a glass and serve immediately.

Nutrition: Calories: 406 Fat: 17.5 g Carbs: 57.3 g Protein: 11.8 g

Banana & Oat Smoothie

Preparation Time: 5 Minutes

Cooking Time: 12 Minutes

Servings: 1

Ingredients:

- 1 banana
- ½ cup unsweetened almond milk
- ¼ cup low-fat Greek yogurt
- ½ cup coconut milk
- ¼ cup rolled oats
- ½ teaspoon vanilla essence
- 1 pinch of cinnamon
- 1 pinch of nutmeg
- ½ maple syrup
- ½ teaspoon liquid sweetener

Directions:

1. Place all the ingredients in the blender and blitz until smooth. Serve immediately.

Nutrition: Calories: 239 Fat: 4 g Carbs: 36 g Protein: 11 g

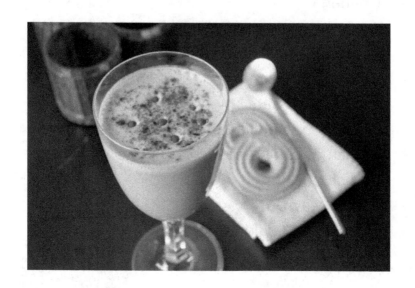

Blueberry, Banana & Chia Smoothie

Preparation Time: 5 Minutes

Cooking Time: 0 Minutes

Servings: 1

Ingredients:

- 2 teaspoon rice protein powder
- ¼ cup frozen banana
- ½ cup low FODMAP milk
- ½ cup blueberries
- ¼ cup vanilla soy ice cream (or lactose-free ice cream or lactose-free yogurt)
- 1 teaspoon chia seeds
- 1 teaspoon lemon juice
- ½ tablespoon maple syrup
- 6 ice cubes

Directions:

1. Place all ingredients in a blender and blitz well. Pour into a serving glass and serve immediately.

Nutrition: Calories: 308 Fat: 10 g Carbs: 50 g Protein: 6 g

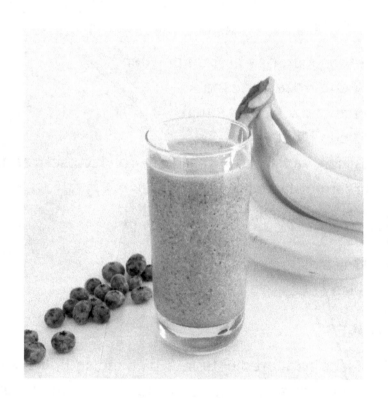

CPSIA information can be obtained
at www.ICGtesting.com
Printed in the USA
BVHW091603190421
605301BV00002B/239

9 781802 331660